Word Retrieval
Practice Pages

Word Exercises for Adults

ISBN: 979-8-987156-2-5

Contents

Contents

Introduction

Word Retrieval

Word retrieval, or word finding, is the process of mentally identifying a word and then verbalizing it. We have all experienced word retrieval difficulties at one time or another; it's that feeling of having a word on the tip of your tongue, but not being able to produce it. For those experiencing the effects of a stroke, brain trauma, disease, or memory loss, these minor instances can become a persistent and frustrating issue. Engaging in word exercises may improve word retrieval skills.

How Words Are Stored

Think of your brain as a filing cabinet. Words are stored systematically, filed away both by sound and meaning. Age, disease, or brain injury may cause your filing cabinet to become rusty, making it harder to gain access to the words you want to use.

This Book

These practice pages aim to grease the tracks of your filing cabinet. With over 2000 target words, these pages provide an opportunity to strengthen the brain's neural pathways by touching upon words known, but not regularly accessed. Items are designed to align with our natural systems for word storage by addressing word relationships, categories, definitions, and word structure. Customizable pages, strategies to use within conversation, and ideas for additional practice are also provided.

Word Retrieval Strategies

Describe It	• Describe the word. Tell what it looks like and how it is used. Provide as many details as possible.
Compare & Contrast	• "It's like a..., but..."
Use Associated Words	• Say any words that come to mind when searching for the word.
Use a Substitute	• Use a word with a similar meaning.
Use Your Hands	• Imitate actions, point, or indicate size and shape.
Draw It	• Keep a notebook handy and draw the word or related objects.
Use the Alphabet	• Go through each letter in your mind. Often a letter will "ring a bell" as being the first letter, making it easier to access.
Take A Break	• Fatigue, distractions, and stress can all impact word retrieval. Take a break and the word may come to you later.

Strategies for Helpers

Help your partner retrieve words by providing cues.

Example: target word = jelly

Provide the category:	*it's a food*
Tell how it is used:	*you spread it*
Provide a rhyming word:	*it rhymes with belly*
Begin a sentence or phrase	*peanut butter and……*
Sound out the first letter:	*j…….*
Sound out additional letters	*jel……..*
Model the name if needed:	*jelly*

CUING IN CONVERSATION

If you notice your partner having trouble finding a word in conversation, remind them to use their strategies.

Be specific. For example, *"Describe it to me."* or *"Can you think of the first letter?"*

Ask yes-no questions until you know the intended word and can provide it for them.

Practice Word List

When you notice a name or word that is repeatedly hard to retrieve, write it below. Add words to the list as you become aware of them. Review daily until the words become easy to access.

_____ _____

_____ _____

_____ _____

_____ _____

_____ _____

_____ _____

_____ _____

_____ _____

Practice Activities

Watch a trivia or game show on TV	• Wheel of Fortune • America Says • Chain Reaction
Play a word board game	• Scrabble • Boggle • Scattegories
Work a word puzzle from a magazine or newspaper	• Crossword Puzzle • Word Search • Jumble
Play a word game app on your phone or tablet	• Word Crush • Wordscapes • 4 Pics 1 Word

Associated Fill-ins

Add vowels to complete words associated with:

CAMPING

1. b __ c k p __ c k

2. t __ n t

3. s t __ r s

4. f __ r __ w __ __ d

5. r __ n g __ r

6. c __ m p s __ t __

7. l __ n t __ r n

8. c __ m p __ s s

9. s l __ __ p __ n g   b __ g

10. s' m __ r __ s

11. b __ n __ c __ l __ r s

12. c __ b __ n

13. h __ m m __ c k

14. b __ n f __ r __

Associated Fill-ins

Add vowels to complete words associated with:

FISHING

1. p __ l __

2. b __ __ t

3. b __ b b __ r

4. h __ __ k

5. s __ n k __ r

6. n __ t

7. t __ c k l __   b __ x

8. l __ r __

9. r __ __ l

10. w __ d __ r s

11. c __ s t

12. r __ v __ r

13. d __ __ p – s __ __

14. r __ d

Associated Fill-ins

Add vowels to complete words associated with:

BOOKS

1. t __ t l __

2. h __ r d c __ v __ r

3. c h __ p t __ r

4. p __ g __ s

5. b __ __ g r __ p h y

6. b __ __ k m __ r k

7. c __ v __ r

8. __ l l __ s t r __ t __ r

9. p __ b l __ s h __ r

10. f __ c t __ __ n

11. b __ __ k w __ r m

12. p __ p __ r b __ c k

13. l __ b r __ r y

14. __ __ t h __ r

Add vowels to complete words associated with:

TRAVEL

1. l __ g g __ g __

2. v __ c __ t __ __ n

3. r __ __ d   t r __ p

4. r __ s __ r v __ t __ __ n

5. t r __ v __ l   __ g __ n t

6. s __ g h t s __ __ __ n g

7. p __ s s p __ r t

8. r __ s t   s t __ p

9. h __ t __ l

10. d __ s t __ n __ t __ __ n

11. r __ s __ r t

12. __ __ r p l __ n __

13. c r __ __ s __   s h __ p

14. t __ __ r __ s t

Associated Fill-ins

Add vowels to complete words associated with:

MONEY

1. d __ ll __ r

2. d __ p __ s __ t

3. ch __ ng __   j __ r

4. b __ n d s

5. __ n t __ r __ s t

6. s t __ c k b r __ k __ r

7. m __ n __ y   __ r d __ r

8. d __ b __ t   c __ r d

9. t r __ n s f __ r

10. c h __ c k __ n g   __ c c __ __ n t

11. w __ t h d r __ w __ l

12. b __ d g __ t

13. s __ v __ n g s

14. w __ __ l t h y

Add vowels to complete words associated with:

WEATHER

1. s __ n n y

2. t h __ n d __ r s t __ r m

3. w __ r m   b r __ __ z __

4. f __ r __ c __ s t

5. h __ m __ d __ t y

6. d r __ z z l __

7. t __ m p __ r __ t __ r __

8. t __ r n __ d __

9. c l __ m __ t __   c h __ n g __

10. s n __ w   f l __ r r __ __ s

11. j __ t   s t r __ __ m

12. b l __ z z __ r d

13. p r __ c __ p __ t __ t __ __ n

14. m __ t __ __ r __ l __ g __ s t

Word Deduction

Determine the word described by each set of clues.

Example: fruit-bunch-wine _____*grapes*_____

1.   animal-tall-neck _____

2.   tool-dig-dirt _____

3.   utensil-bowl-soup _____

4.   game-piece-roll _____

5.   greens-dressing-tossed _____

6.   spider-silk-spin _____

7.   egg-center-yellow _____

8.   beard-shave-blade _____

9.   ride-three-wheels _____

10. window-hanging-fabric _____

11. tool-chop-wood _____

12. fruit-yellow-peel _____

13. bird-arctic-tuxedo _____

14. cat-vibrating-sound _____

15. eat-outdoor-basket _____

Word Deduction

Determine the word described by each set of clues.

Example: fruit-bunch-wine   _____ *grapes* _____

1. pancake-topping-maple   _____

2. bird-fly-flap   _____

3. coach-blow-loud   _____

4. animal-tentacles-eight   _____

5. string-teeth-clean   _____

6. walk-steady-stick   _____

7. appliance-carpet-suction   _____

8. bread-edge-hard   _____

9. number-twelve-eggs   _____

10. house-storage-above   _____

11. animal-spray-odor   _____

12. dog-walk-rope   _____

13. cook-charcoal-grate   _____

14. music-keys-bench   _____

15. water-tube-garden   _____

Word Deduction

Determine the word described by each set of clues.

Example: fruit-bunch-wine   _grapes_

1. pencil-topper-pink   _____

2. plant-desert-spiny   _____

3. turtle-covering-hard   _____

4. wall-color-brush   _____

5. royal-head-jewels   _____

6. skin-permanent-ink   _____

7. animal-forest-quills   _____

8. ring-sparkle-carat   _____

9. kangaroo-joey-carry   _____

10. store-checkout-worker   _____

11. historical-stone-figure   _____

12. animal-desert-hump   _____

13. baseball-team-shelter   _____

14. metal-attract-refrigerator   _____

15. daily-capsule-nutrition   _____

Word Deduction

Determine the word described by each set of clues.

Example: fruit-bunch-wine _____*grapes*_____

1. sleep-soft-head _____

2. gum-blow-pop _____

3. truck-snow-remove _____

4. roof-brick-smokestack _____

5. child-payment-chores _____

6. dog-neck-tags _____

7. knight-protection-shiny _____

8. foot-bottom-curve _____

9. chemical-sanitize-whiten _____

10. shopping-metal-buggy _____

11. sleep-noise-nose _____

12. rubber-inflate-helium _____

13. profession-airplane-fly _____

14. words-definitions-book _____

15. wedding-annual-celebrate _____

Word Deduction

Determine the word described by each set of clues.

Example: fruit-bunch-wine _____grapes_____

1. car-yellow-fare _____

2. country-symbol-fabric _____

3. church-walkway-bride _____

4. king-royal-chair _____

5. volcano-red-hot _____

6. college-money-award _____

7. stretch-pose-mat _____

8. puppies-birth-group _____

9. metal-lightweight-can _____

10. coffee-ingredient-stimulant _____

11. teeth-artificial-removeable _____

12. snake-substance-poison _____

13. tropical-storm-wind _____

14. grass-single-strand _____

15. basketball-steady-bounce _____

Words That Follow

Think of a word or phrase that might follow the given word.

Ex: pony ___tail___ ___Express___

1. hot _____ _____

2. shopping _____ _____

3. sweet _____ _____

4. book _____ _____

5. dish _____ _____

6. good _____ _____

7. tea _____ _____

8. chicken _____ _____

9. sea _____ _____

10. mail _____ _____

11. tooth _____ _____

12. rain _____ _____

13. vanilla _____ _____

14. beach _____ _____

Words That Follow

Think of a word or phrase that might follow the given word.

Ex: pony   _____tail_____   _____Express_____

1.   ice   _____   _____

2.   fried   _____   _____

3.   lucky   _____   _____

4.   weather   _____   _____

5.   eye   _____   _____

6.   water   _____   _____

7.   car   _____   _____

8.   tomato   _____   _____

9.   bath   _____   _____

10. coffee   _____   _____

11. silver   _____   _____

12. heart   _____   _____

13. fortune   _____   _____

14. apple   _____   _____

Words That Follow

Think of a word or phrase that might follow the given word.

Ex: pony   _____tail_____   _____Express_____

1. best   _____   _____

2. tree   _____   _____

3. pork   _____   _____

4. sand   _____   _____

5. snow   _____   _____

6. shredded   _____   _____

7. window   _____   _____

8. night   _____   _____

9. potato   _____   _____

10. salad   _____   _____

11. hair   _____   _____

12. pillow   _____   _____

13. gold   _____   _____

14. hula   _____   _____

Words That Follow

Think of a word or phrase that might follow the given word.

Ex: pony   _____tail_____   _____Express_____

1. bird   _____   _____

2. honey   _____   _____

3. cotton   _____   _____

4. life   _____   _____

5. lunch   _____   _____

6. gift   _____   _____

7. wind   _____   _____

8. house   _____   _____

9. ear   _____   _____

10. dirty   _____   _____

11. middle   _____   _____

12. rocking   _____   _____

13. sun   _____   _____

14. belly   _____   _____

Listing Associated Words

List words associated with each location.

a forest

_____ _____ _____

_____ _____ _____

_____ _____ _____

a farm

_____ _____ _____

_____ _____ _____

_____ _____ _____

a beach

_____ _____ _____

_____ _____ _____

_____ _____ _____

Listing Associated Words

List words associated with each location.

a baseball game

_____ _____ _____

_____ _____ _____

_____ _____ _____

a wedding

_____ _____ _____

_____ _____ _____

_____ _____ _____

a circus

_____ _____ _____

_____ _____ _____

_____ _____ _____

Listing Associated Words

List words associated with each location.

a school

_____   _____   _____

_____   _____   _____

_____   _____   _____

an airport

_____   _____   _____

_____   _____   _____

_____   _____   _____

a nursery

_____   _____   _____

_____   _____   _____

_____   _____   _____

Scrambled Categories

Unscramble the letters to form items in each category.
The first letter has been underlined.

TYPES OF BREAD

1. E R Y   _____

2. L E O H W   T W A H E   _____

3. T I P A   _____

4. R N O C   _____

5. M P U P R E N E C K I L   _____

6. N A B A A N   _____

7. S D H G U O O U R   _____

TYPES OF CAKE

1. T U R F I C K A E   _____

2. D R E   T E V V L E   _____

3. G A E L N   D O F O   _____

4. C O H L T E C A O   _____

5. S E E E H C A E K C   _____

6. T O A R R C   _____

7. E L O N M   _____

Scrambled Categories

Unscramble the letters to form items in each category.
The first letter has been underlined.

TYPES OF MUSIC

1. Z A J Z   _____

2. D C I S O   _____

3. O R C K & L R L O _____

4. K L F O   _____

5. Y R C U T N O   _____

6. H I P   P O H   _____

7. C L S S A C A I L _____

TYPES OF DANCE

1. A P T   _____

2. R O B L L A O M _____

3. T L E B A L   _____

4. O K L P A   _____

5. N C A - N C A   _____

6. T G A N O   _____

7. Y O H E K   Y O P E K _____

Scrambled Categories

Unscramble the letters to form items in each category.
The first letter has been underlined.

TYPES OF SHOES

1. Y N E <u>P</u> N <u>L</u> F O A R E _____

2. O L G <u>C</u> _____

3. <u>S</u> A D L A N _____

4. R K E E A <u>S</u> N _____

5. <u>F</u> I L P – L O P <u>F</u> _____

6. <u>H</u> H G I L <u>H</u> E E _____

7. <u>C</u> W O O B Y T O <u>B</u> O _____

TYPES OF FABRIC

1. L I <u>S</u> K _____

2. O L O <u>W</u> _____

3. V S N <u>C</u> A A _____

4. P L A <u>B</u> R U _____

5. <u>N</u> Y L N O _____

6. O <u>C</u> T T O N _____

7. <u>P</u> O E Y S E T L R _____

Scrambled Categories

Unscramble the letters to form items in each category.
The first letter has been underlined.

TYPES OF TRUCKS

1. M E <u>S</u> I   _____

2. U P M <u>D</u>   _____

3. O W <u>T</u>   _____

4. <u>C</u> E E M T N   _____

5. <u>G</u> B R A G E A   _____

6. U K <u>P</u> P C I   _____

7. <u>D</u> V Y E I E L R   _____

TYPES OF BOATS

1. G U <u>T</u> B T O A   _____

2. N <u>C</u> O A E   _____

3. T H <u>Y</u> C A   _____

4. I <u>S</u> L A B T O A   _____

5. Y R <u>F</u> R E   _____

6. <u>S</u> E D E P B T O A   _____

7. A R G <u>B</u> E   _____

Scrambled Categories

Unscramble the letters to form items in each category.
The first letter has been underlined.

COUNTRIES

1. I D R E L N A   _____

2. Z A B I R L   _____

3. R O M O O C C   _____

4. N R A W O Y   _____

5. O P L N A D   _____

6. Z I W S T E R A L N D   _____

7. P Y G E T   _____

LANGUAGES

1. I I L A A T N   _____

2. N E F C H R   _____

3. S H I E N G L   _____

4. P G O U R T S E E U   _____

5. K E E R G   _____

6. E S E N C H I   _____

7. N S I G G A N U L A G E   _____

Scrambled Categories

Unscramble the letters to form items in each category.
The first letter has been underlined.

PLANETS

1. C R Y U <u>M</u> E R   _____

2. S N U <u>V</u> E   _____

3. T A R H <u>E</u>   _____

4. R E <u>J</u> U P I T   _____

5. <u>N</u> P E U N T E   _____

6. N U R T A <u>S</u>   _____

7. S R <u>M</u> A   _____

TABLE OF ELEMENTS

1. P P <u>C</u> O E R   _____

2. B R A <u>C</u> O N   _____

3. <u>N</u> R O I T G E N   _____

4. D I <u>S</u> O U M   _____

5. Y E X <u>O</u> G N   _____

6. R O N <u>I</u>   _____

7. E N G O R D Y <u>H</u>   _____

ANIMALS

Think of an animal that begins with each letter of the alphabet.

A _____   J _____   S _____

B _____   K _____   T _____

C _____   L _____   U _nicorn_____

D _____   M _____   V _____

E _____   N _____   W _____

F _____   O _____   X _-ray fish_____

G _____   P _____   Y _____

H _____   Q _____   Z _____

I _____   R _____

FOODS

Think of a food that begins with each letter of the alphabet.

A _____   J_____   S _____

B _____   K _____   T _____

C _____   L _____   U _pside-down cake___

D _____   M_____   V _____

E _____   N _____   W _____

F _____   O _____   X _-mas cookies_____

G _____   P _____   Y _____

H _____   Q_____   Z _iti pasta_____

I _____   R _____

Categories A-Z

WOMEN'S NAMES

Think of a woman's name that begins with each letter of the alphabet.

A _____

B _____

C _____

D _____

E _____

F _____

G _____

H _____

I _____

J _____

K _____

L _____

M _____

N _____

O _____

P _____

Q uinn _____

R _____

S _____

T _____

U rsula _____

V _____

W _____

X ena _____

Y _____

Z elda _____

Categories A-Z

MEN'S NAMES

Think of a man's name that begins with each letter of the alphabet.

A _____   J _____   S _____

B _____   K _____   T _____

C _____   L _____   U _lysses_____

D _____   M _____   V _____

E _____   N _____   W _____

F _____   O _____   X _avier_____

G _____   P _____   Y _anni_____

H _____   Q _____   Z _____

I _____   R _____

Categories by Letter

Think of an item in each category that starts with the given letter.

A

City _____

State _____

Country _____

School Subject _____

Occupation _____

Body Part _____

Tree _____

Vegetable _____

Nut _____

Type of Pie _____

B

City _____

School Subject _____

Car Part _____

Dog Breed _____

Fish _____

Card Game _____

Sport _____

Vegetable _____

Breakfast Food _____

Type of Pie _____

Word Retrieval
Practice Pages

35

Copyright 2023
J. Perkins Press

Categories by Letter

Think of an item in each category that starts with the given letter.

C

City _____

Dog Breed _____

Bird _____

Fish _____

Flower _____

Beverage _____

Nut _____

Spice _____

Type of Pie _____

Ice Cream Flavor _____

D

City _____

State _____

Country _____

Occupation _____

Dog Breed _____

Tree _____

Flower _____

Gemstone _____

Breakfast Food _____

Spice _____

Categories by Letter

Think of an item in each category that starts with the given letter.

E

City _____

Country _____

Occupation _____

Body Part _____

Car Part _____

Bird _____

Fish _____

Tree _____

Gemstone _____

Vegetable _____

F

City _____

State _____

Country _____

Holiday _____

Occupation _____

Body Part _____

Car Part _____

Bird _____

Fish _____

Sport _____

Categories by Letter

Think of an item in each category that starts with the given letter.

G	**H**
State _____	City _____
Country _____	State _____
School Subject _____	Country _____
Occupation _____	School Subject _____
Body Part _____	Occupation _____
Dog Breed _____	Car Part _____
Fish _____	Bird _____
Sport _____	Sport _____
Fruit _____	Musical Instrument _____
Spice _____	Nut _____

Categories by Letter

Think of an item in each category that starts with the given letter.

I	K
City _____	City _____
State _____	State _____
Country _____	Country _____
Color _____	Color _____
Occupation _____	Body Part _____
Body Part _____	Sport _____
Car Part _____	Musical Instrument _____
Flower _____	Card Game _____
Beverage _____	Fruit _____
Type of Pie _____	Vegetable _____

Word Retrieval
Practice Pages

Copyright 2023
J. Perkins Press

Categories by Letter

Think of an item in each category that starts with the given letter.

L

City _____

State _____

Holiday _____

Color _____

Occupation _____

Dog Breed _____

Flower _____

Fruit_____

Vegetable _____

Beverage _____

M

City _____

State _____

Holiday _____

Color _____

Occupation _____

Fish _____

Flower _____

Fruit_____

Nut_____

Ice Cream Flavor _____

Categories by Letter

Think of an item in each category that starts with the given letter.

N

City _____

State _____

Country _____

Holiday _____

Color _____

Occupation _____

Body Part _____

Fruit_____

Spice _____

Ice Cream Flavor _____

O

City _____

State _____

Occupation _____

Bird _____

Tree _____

Gemstone _____

Musical Instrument_____

Fruit_____

Vegetable _____

Breakfast Food _____

Categories by Letter

Think of an item in each category that starts with the given letter.

P

Dog Breed _____

Bird _____

Tree_____

Gemstone _____

Musical Instrument _____

Card Game _____

Breakfast Food _____

Nut _____

Spice _____

Type of Pie _____

R

State _____

Occupation _____

Bird _____

Tree _____

Flower _____

Gemstone _____

Card Game _____

Fruit_____

Vegetable _____

Beverage _____

Categories by Letter

Think of an item in each category that starts with the given letter.

S	**T**
State _____	City _____
School Subject _____	State _____
Occupation _____	Holiday _____
Dog Breed _____	Color _____
Bird _____	Occupation _____
Flower _____	Body Part_____
Sport _____	Car Part _____
Musical Instrument _____	Dog Breed _____
Card Game _____	Bird _____
Ice Cream Flavor _____	Spice _____

Categories by Letter

Think of an item in each category that starts with the given letter.

V

City _____

State _____

Country _____

Holiday _____

Occupation _____

Bird _____

Flower _____

Sport _____

Musical Instrument _____

Ice Cream Flavor _____

W

City _____

State _____

Occupation _____

Body Part_____

Car Part _____

Bird _____

Tree _____

Fruit_____

Breakfast Food _____

Nut_____

Listing Category Members

List items in each category.

THINGS THAT ARE GREEN

_____

_____

_____

_____

_____

_____

THINGS THAT ARE YELLOW

_____

_____

_____

_____

_____

_____

Listing Category Members

List items in each category.

KITCHEN UTENSILS	**SWEET TREATS**
_____	_____
_____	_____
_____	_____
_____	_____
_____	_____
_____	_____
_____	_____

Listing Category Members

List items in each category.

TOOLS   **BUGS**

_____   _____

_____   _____

_____   _____

_____   _____

_____   _____

_____   _____

_____   _____

Listing Category Members

List items in each category.

SPORTS TEAMS	FAMOUS LANDMARKS
_____	_____
_____	_____
_____	_____
_____	_____
_____	_____
_____	_____
_____	_____

A

1. a weight used to hold a ship   _____

2. someone who plays a role in a movie   _____

3. a garment worn when cooking   _____

4. a photo storage book   _____

5. the nut of an oak tree   _____

6. clapping that expresses approval   _____

7. a gymnast   _____

8. the remains of a fire   _____

9. not in attendance   _____

10. the gas pedal in a car   _____

11. the science of farming   _____

12. to respect and look up to   _____

13. a loud fire warning   _____

14. a strong, pleasant smell   _____

B

1. an eye movement _____

2. a sweeping tool _____

3. wrist jewelry _____

4. an unmarried man _____

5. having an unsweet taste _____

6. a drinkable liquid _____

7. to burp loudly _____

8. able to speak two languages _____

9. a large bundle of hay _____

10. a person with brown hair _____

11. a witch's liquid concoction _____

12. the card used to cast a vote _____

13. a throwing object that returns _____

14. to stand on one foot _____

C

1. a hair-grooming tool   _____

2. a child's drawing utensil   _____

3. the raised edge of a street   _____

4. the last car of a train   _____

5. a person who tells jokes for a living   _____

6. an edible ice cream holder   _____

7. a book of items for purchase   _____

8. self-assured   _____

9. a small fragment of bread or cookie   _____

10. to end a membership or subscription   _____

11. to travel to and from work   _____

12. the pilot's area of a plane   _____

13. a discount clipped from the paper   _____

14. a broken arm protector   _____

D

1. a powerful explosive   _____

2. to vanish   _____

3. an assistant sheriff   _____

4. a period of ten years   _____

5. a barrier preventing water flow   _____

6. to process food in the colon   _____

7. a dark, underground prison   _____

8. to give to charity   _____

9. an alternate route   _____

10. a college residence hall   _____

11. to distribute playing cards   _____

12. a private journal   _____

13. a mythical fire-breathing creature   _____

14. a sandwich shop   _____

	Begins With	

E

1. repeated sound waves   _____

2. to secretly marry   _____

3. moving stairs   _____

4. to go into a building   _____

5. creepy   _____

6. to sign up for classes   _____

7. an animal that no longer exists   _____

8. suitable for eating   _____

9. to secretly listen   _____

10. a political contest   _____

11. to breathe out   _____

12. a mistake   _____

13. to flee from a dangerous situation _____

14. the main course of a meal   _____

F

1. pigmented skin spots   _____

2. an elevated body temperature   _____

3. the burst of light from a camera   _____

4. the one that is liked the most   _____

5. a game played with a dog   _____

6. to break, as a bone   _____

7. a water spout   _____

8. occurring often   _____

9. to drop a football   _____

10. acquainted with   _____

11. to attach, as a seatbelt   _____

12. a house heater   _____

13. someone running from the law   _____

14. an out of bounds baseball   _____

G

1. a large, hard swallow   _____

2. a prison watchman   _____

3. to wager money in a casino   _____

4. a place where art is exhibited   _____

5. a turkey's sound   _____

6. a visitor in one's home   _____

7. not brand name   _____

8. a lighthearted laugh   _____

9. to assure quality   _____

10. a round model of the earth   _____

11. a spirit that lives in the bottle   _____

12. soccer scoring zone   _____

13. a sudden rush of wind   _____

14. the rules of language   _____

Begins With

H

1. a horse's foot   _____

2. events in the past   _____

3. a laundry basket   _____

4. to be truthful   _____

5. to produce a tune without words   _____

6. a safe port for boats   _____

7. a daily behavior   _____

8. the aura circling an angel   _____

9. a bumblebee's home   _____

10. modest   _____

11. to sleep through the winter   _____

12. a door joint   _____

13. a small outdoor shack   _____

14. a track and field obstacle   _____

Begins With

I

1. a deep blue color _____

2. against the law _____

3. not susceptible to disease _____

4. a list of page numbers _____

5. to fill with air _____

6. to mimic _____

7. a dome made of snow _____

8. to set on fire _____

9. money earned _____

10. not guilty _____

11. having the same features, as twins _____

12. to completely disregard _____

13. a person posing as someone else _____

14. an elephant's tusk _____

J

1.   a lightweight coat   _____

2.   to toss multiple balls in the air   _____

3.   a dried meat snack   _____

4.   a funny statement   _____

5.   a high-powered plane   _____

6.   denim pants   _____

7.   a group that delivers a verdict   _____

8.   a tropical forest   _____

9.   a large, leopard-like cat   _____

10.   envious of another   _____

11.   the wild card in a deck   _____

12.   to run slowly   _____

13.   an adolescent   _____

14.   a coin-operated music machine   _____

Begins With

K

1. the class before first grade _____

2. a form of self-defense _____

3. a flying toy _____

4. a pleated skirt worn in Scotland _____

5. body organs that filter waste _____

6. a small Australian bear _____

7. a small plastic boat _____

8. a barrel used to store beer _____

9. a pot used to boil water _____

10. a dog cage _____

11. a small piece of corn _____

12. a computer's typing accessory _____

13. fuel for an oil lamp _____

14. finger joints _____

L

1. a long, luxurious car   _____

2. a soft, twisted candy   _____

3. lacking motivation   _____

4. the words to a song   _____

5. where water escapes from a pipe   _____

6. a deep spoon with a long handle   _____

7. a waiting room   _____

8. a looped rope for catching cattle   _____

9. money borrowed from the bank   _____

10. a company's trademark   _____

11. to send a rocket into space   _____

12. a soft white cooking fat   _____

13. to create foam with shampoo   _____

14. a sleep-time song   _____

M

1. upper lip hair   _____

2. a list of food options   _____

3. to use a ruler   _____

4. a baseball glove   _____

5. a small glass ball   _____

6. an elected town leader   _____

7. a large wall painting   _____

8. to knead muscles   _____

9. livestock waste   _____

10. a large, disorderly group   _____

11. to soak meat in sauce   _____

12. a daytime performance   _____

13. a shopping center   _____

14. a fine cloud of water   _____

Word Retrieval
Practice Pages

61

N

1. loud
    _____

2. tortilla chips and cheese
    _____

3. a bright, fluorescent color
    _____

4. a mesh butterfly trap
    _____

5. a child's caregiver
    _____

6. slender in width
    _____

7. a bad dream
    _____

8. to take small bites
    _____

9. neither positive nor negative
    _____

10. a solid lump of gold
    _____

11. spaghetti and lo mein, for example
    _____

12. unable to feel
    _____

13. to propose a candidate for office
    _____

14. sweet juice from fruits and flowers
    _____

O

1. a solemn promise _____

2. an egg shape _____

3. a room where paperwork is done _____

4. a particular smell _____

5. easily discovered _____

6. a large, flightless bird _____

7. a thick, topical medicine _____

8. overweight _____

9. a musical drama _____

10. the first, often copied _____

11. a large group of musicians _____

12. internal body parts _____

13. a collection of fruit trees _____

14. a person who is hopeful for the future _____

Begins With

P

1.   a small pool of rainwater _____

2.   a royal home _____

3.   to trim branches from a tree _____

4.   a bird found in city parks _____

5.   to row a canoe _____

6.   a pleasant, bottled scent _____

7.   colorful fingernail gloss _____

8.   where convicted felons live _____

9.   a cucumber preserved in brine _____

10.   allergy-producing plant dust _____

11.   to puncture holes in one's earlobes _____

12.   a hooded arctic coat _____

13.   to remove the skin of a fruit _____

14.   to squeeze one's cheeks _____

	Begins With

Q

1. to resign   _____

2. a small game bird   _____

3. to ask   _____

4. ¼ gallon   _____

5. to satisfy one's thirst   _____

6. nauseated   _____

7. a short test   _____

8. isolation following illness   _____

9. a patchwork blanket   _____

10. an egg pie   _____

11. happening every 3 months   _____

12. an earth tremor   _____

13. to cite another's words   _____

14. simple and old fashioned   _____

R

1.   tennis equipment   _____

2.   to fix   _____

3.   a baby's noisy toy   _____

4.   a cold-blooded vertebrate   _____

5.   to practice a performance   _____

6.   spoiled   _____

7.   an allergic skin reaction   _____

8.   to save from danger   _____

9.   a long-barreled firearm   _____

10.   cooking instructions   _____

11.   an annual family gathering   _____

12.   to clean with water   _____

13.   a list of job experience   _____

14.   a bath coat   _____

S

1.   a list of appointments _____

2.   a neck warmer _____

3.   a cast iron frying pan _____

4.   the absence of noise _____

5.   a hunting expedition _____

6.   a wetland _____

7.   material that smooths wood _____

8.   ½ of a school year _____

9.   the mist from hot water _____

10. annual income _____

11. evidence of a prior skin cut _____

12. a free trial of a product _____

13. overlapping roof tiles _____

14. a hanging arm bandage _____

T

1. a drop from an eye   _____

2. a pub   _____

3. to warm from frozen   _____

4. to tell on someone   _____

5. natural ability   _____

6. a military vehicle   _____

7. porcelain flooring   _____

8. a partial wig   _____

9. a 2-year-old   _____

10. a statue given to the winner   _____

11. vehicle congestion   _____

12. men's formalwear   _____

13. a cigarette leaf   _____

14. sworn statements to the court   _____

Begins With

U

1.   a kitchen tool   _____

2.   a sports official   _____

3.   calling for immediate action   _____

4.   military or sports clothing   _____

5.   to grasp the meaning of   _____

6.   one who escorts you to your seat   _____

7.   the entire galaxy   _____

8.   a small, stringed instrument   _____

9.   an academic institution   _____

10.   provides protection from the rain   _____

11.   an ideally perfect place   _____

12.   distinctive; one of a kind   _____

13.   to cover a chair with fabric   _____

14.   a decision where all are in agreement   _____

V

1. eyesight   _____

2. a thick, smooth fabric   _____

3. a small, rural community   _____

4. the level of noise   _____

5. the highest-ranking student   _____

6. a bride's face covering   _____

7. conceited   _____

8. a parking attendant   _____

9. a protective furniture glaze   _____

10. a sour cooking liquid   _____

11. a jury's decision   _____

12. bony segments of the spine   _____

13. a machine that dispenses snacks   _____

14. to vote against a legislative bill   _____

Begins With

W

1. to speak softly   _____

2. an entire collection of clothing   _____

3. a magician's tool   _____

4. a tool used for twisting a bolt   _____

5. to use more than necessary   _____

6. a large storage building   _____

7. a wire mixing utensil   _____

8. an open injury   _____

9. a ballroom dance   _____

10. to become limp, as a flower   _____

11. a document authorizing arrest   _____

12. a round door decoration   _____

13. knowledge from life experience   _____

14. to step through water   _____

Y

1. a sweet potato _____

2. a bread ingredient _____

3. knitting fiber _____

4. a 3-foot measuring tool _____

5. to pull quickly and vigorously _____

6. a long-haired ox _____

7. to give way in traffic _____

8. an ape-like creature from folklore _____

9. annually _____

10. a creamy dairy product _____

11. young people _____

12. to long for _____

13. to bark snappishly _____

14. to sing with rapid changes in pitch _____

Z

1. a summer squash   _____

2. a state of peace and calm   _____

3. a pimple   _____

4. a metal clothing fastener   _____

5. an essential nutrient   _____

6. a brightly colored flower   _____

7. the study of animals   _____

8. a suspended harness ride   _____

9. to move back and forth sharply   _____

10. a specific area   _____

11. the twelve astrological signs   _____

12. one minus one   _____

13. a type of sandwich bag closure   _____

14. kooky, like a clown   _____

Wh- Definitions

What.....

1. is a baby's chin cloth? _____

2. is a Hawaiian feast? _____

3. is the cord in a candle? _____

4. is the front of your lower leg? _____

5. is a vessel that travels under water? _____

6. are elastic straps that hold up pants? _____

7. is a hand-controlled doll? _____

8. is the heartbeat felt in your wrist? _____

9. is a tight clump in a shoelace? _____

10. is loose rock on a country road? _____

11. is the bill of a bird? _____

12. is a graduation certificate? _____

13. is a mountain snowslide? _____

14. is a school milk container? _____

Wh- Definitions

What.....

1. is a football headpiece? _____

2. is an ornamental water spout?_____

3. is a coat without sleeves?_____

4. is raw cake mix? _____

5. are the colored segments of a flower? _____

6. are the wood chunks in a campfire? _____

7. is a sale where items are bid on? _____

8. is a rod that detects TV signals? _____

9. is a person's desire to eat?_____

10. is an electronic math device? _____

11. is an insulated coffee jug? _____

12. is the substance that stiffens clothing? _____

13. is the force that pulls us to the earth?_____

14. is the number sequence that opens lock? _____

Wh- Definitions

Who.....

1. is the leader of a ship? _____

2. gives a shave and a haircut? _____

3. plays music on the radio? _____

4. fills and monitors prescriptions? _____

5. completes tax forms? _____

6. drives a limousine? _____

7. is the leader of a school? _____

8. shows local sites to travelers? _____

9. sews clothing? _____

10. is a private teacher? _____

11. rides in a horse race? _____

12. monitors a swimming pool? _____

13. gets paid to play professional sports? _____

14. fills in when the teacher is away? _____

Wh- Definitions

Who.....

1. creates flower arrangements? _____

2. shows homes for sale? _____

3. cleans a school? _____

4. treats skin conditions? _____

5. draws pictures in storybooks? _____

6. designs buildings? _____

7. leads an orchestra? _____

8. donates time to a worthy cause? _____

9. sprays for pests? _____

10. adjusts the spine? _____

11. extracts coal or gold? _____

12. creates their own company? _____

13. creates dance routines? _____

14. provides food service for large events? _____

Wh- Definitions

Where.....

1. do students eat? _____

2. are dry food items stored? _____

3. do homeless pets live? _____

4. do judges hear cases? _____

5. are coin-operated washers used? _____

6. are school plays held? _____

7. do acrobats and animal trainers perform? _____

8. is money stored within a bank? _____

9. do scientists conduct experiments? _____

10. do people play slots and poker? _____

11. are horses kept on a farm? _____

12. are movies shown? _____

13. are fish and sea life on display? _____

14. are football games held? _____

Wh- Definitions

Where.....

1. do musicians record their work? _____

2. are products mass produced? _____

3. do athletes dress for a game? _____

4. is wine stored? _____

5. are bread and cookies sold? _____

6. do seedlings grow in the winter? _____

7. are dogs washed and trimmed? _____

8. are tent sites reserved? _____

9. do chickens live on a farm? _____

10. do people go to roller skate? _____

11. do people place a vote? _____

12. are airplanes stored at the airport? _____

13. is grain stored? _____

14. do people play pinball and video games? _____

Double Definitions

Think of a word that fits both definitions.

Ex.   a nocturnal bird/baseball equipment _____*bat*_____

1.   a golf stick/a stacked sandwich _____

2.   a large pebble/to sway back and forth _____

3.   to organize papers/a fingernail shaper _____

4.   a tree covering/a dog's cry _____

5.   a journey/to stumble _____

6.   number on a calendar/a dried fruit _____

7.   to frolic/a school performance_____

8.   a gold band/a telephone sound _____

9.   to press with heat/a metal _____

10.   a tin soup container/to be able to _____

11.   to propel with oars/items in a line _____

12.   a person under medical care/to be tolerant _____

Double Definitions

Think of a word that fits both definitions.

Ex.   a nocturnal bird/baseball equipment _____bat_____

1.   spare coins/to transform _____

2.   a horse booth/to delay _____

3.   a channel changer/secluded_____

4.   not wrong/a privilege _____

5.   a place for stray dogs/a unit of weight _____

6.   to put in a secret place/an animal skin _____

7.   to position a car/a city playground _____

8.   a small, round bread/to somersault_____

9.   a gestural greeting/an ocean swell _____

10.   to spar in a ring/a moving container _____

11.   a hair accessory/a hunting weapon _____

12.   to throw a baseball/the slope of a roof _____

Double Definitions

Think of a word that fits both definitions.

Ex.　a nocturnal bird/baseball equipment _____*bat*_____

1.　a tropical tree/part of a hand _____

2.　not yours/to extract gold _____

3.　to form a bow/an equal score _____

4.　a painter's tool/to smooth hair _____

5.　to ignite a fire/not heavy _____

6.　a timepiece/to view _____

7.　a lock opener/a map legend _____

8.　to go first in volleyball/to work in the military _____

9.　number two in line/a small unit of time _____

10.　a rubber wheel/to fatigue _____

11.　a tree limb/a governmental division _____

12.　a college diploma/a measure of temperature _____

Double Definitions

Think of a word that fits both definitions.

Ex.   a nocturnal bird/baseball equipment _____bat_____

1.   jelly/a predicament_____

2.   a crunchy potato snack/a nick _____

3.   a locomotive/to teach _____

4.   talked/part of a bicycle wheel _____

5.   a grizzly/to carry a load_____

6.   men's business wear/similar playing cards _____

7.   a wintergreen flavor/where money is made _____

8.   the swiftest part of a stream/most recent_____

9.   autumn season/to tumble to the ground _____

10.   a weight-tracking tool/a set of musical notes_____

11.   a measuring stick/person in political power _____

12.   blades that rotate air/an enthusiastic spectator _____

Double Definitions

Think of a word that fits both definitions.

Ex.   a nocturnal bird/baseball equipment _____bat_____

1.   a spinning toy/the summit _____

2.   burning flames/to terminate an employee _____

3.   a financial institution/a steep slope _____

4.   a handwashing basin/to drop to the ocean floor _____

5.   a piece of wood/a group of directors_____

6.   to secure an envelope/a sea animal _____

7.   a mallard/to dodge _____

8.   set of employees/a shepherd's rod _____

9.   an uninteresting person/to drill _____

10.   a long storybook/new and unique _____

11.   a corn stem/to relentlessly pursue _____

12.   a skin growth/a burrowing animal _____

Compound Definitions

The two answers will form a new word.

Ex.   365 days + bound pages = a high school memento

    year + book = yearbook

1.   the opposite of down + the rhythm of a song = cheerful

    _____

2.   evening + an elegant dress = sleepwear

    _____

3.   a chewing piece + to lose hold of = a sugar-coated candy

    _____

4.   laid by a chicken + to sow seeds = a colorful vegetable

    _____

5.   a cereal beverage + to jiggle = blended ice cream

    _____

6.   precipitation + a hair accessory = a colorful arc

    _____

7.   bees' nectar + morning mist = a type of melon

    _____

8.   sun's opposite + to polish shoes = homemade alcohol

    _____

Compound Definitions

The two answers will form a new word.

Ex.   365 days + bound pages = a high school memento

year + book = yearbook

1.   granted by a genie + a skeleton piece = good luck when broken

   _____

2.   coarse to the touch + a home = to wrestle

   _____

3.   the organ that pumps blood + to be on fire = reflux

   _____

4.   the opposite of on + the season of blooms = one's children

   _____

5.   large in size + artificial hair = an important person

   _____

6.   an invoice to be paid + a plank of wood = a large ad

   _____

7.   the season of snow + a shade of emerald = a minty flavor

   _____

8.   to ice a cake + a wound from a bug = frozen skin

   _____

Compound Definitions

The two answers will form a new word.

Ex.   365 days + bound pages = a high school memento

year + book = yearbook

1.   to beat wings + a tire changing device = a pancake

   _____

2.   to illustrate + a road over water = a castle entry

   _____

3.   the middle point + a portion of pie = a table decoration

   _____

4.   to fracture + the opposite of slow = the morning meal

   _____

5.   a small steel sewing tool + the tip of a pencil = embroidery

   _____

6.   an auto + to leave = freight

   _____

7.   frog's cousin + a bar seat = a mushroom

   _____

8.   to jump + a type of whiskey = an outdoor children's game

   _____

Compound Definitions

The two answers will form a new word.

Ex.   365 days + bound pages = a high school memento

year + book = yearbook

1.   to burst a balloon + maize = a movie snack

_____

2.   sky-colored + to produce a newspaper = an architect's plans

_____

3.   inexpensive + to glide on ice with bladed shoes = a tightwad

_____

4.   an automobile + a swimming basin = a ride share

_____

5.   a cooking kettle + a pumpkin pastry = a comfort food

_____

6.   to quiet a child + a young dog = a seafood side dish

_____

7.   the opposite of out + sound from vocal cords = an itemized list

_____

8.   a lively Irish dance + a wood-cutting tool = a type of puzzle

_____

The two answers will form a new word.

Ex.   365 days + bound pages = a high school memento

_____year + book = yearbook_____

1. a 25¢ coin + the rear of a building = a football position

    _____

2. sleeping furniture + to cover with jam = a comforter

    _____

3. the opposite of before + arithmetic = an unintended result

    _____

4.   a row of bushes + a pig = a small, spiny animal

    _____

5. to barter + a blemish = a logo

    _____

6. below + a horse-drawn buggy = a car's framework

    _____

7. golf ball warning + to throw a fishing line = weather prediction

    _____

8. to ground a plane + a British nobleman = an apartment owner

    _____

Compound Definitions

The two answers will form a new word.

Ex.   365 days + bound pages = a high school memento

year + book = yearbook

1.   wax and a wick + the opposite of dark = a romantic dinner

   _____

2.   one who inherits the throne + a weaving frame = a keepsake

   _____

3.   not fresh + a life companion = a standoff

   _____

4.   a container for plants + good fortune = a group meal

   _____

5.   to mix playing cards + a piece of lumber = a leisure activity

   _____

6.   to frighten + a large black bird = a garden protector

   _____

7.   a mending fabric + to perform a task for pay = a type of quilt

   _____

8.   theater platform + a sports instructor = a horse-drawn carriage

   _____

Rhyming Definitions

The answers will be two rhyming words.

Ex.   overweight feline   *fat cat*

1.   ancient bacterial growth   _____

2.   indigo footwear   _____

3.   costless maple   _____

4.   enjoyable religious sister   _____

5.   snail-paced black bird   _____

6.   frigid riches   _____

7.   moist tabletop light   _____

8.   tidy empress   _____

9.   dim tree covering   _____

10. speedy tongue swipe   _____

11. authentic sea animal   _____

12. crimson bunk   _____

Rhyming Definitions

The answers will be two rhyming words.

Ex.   overweight feline   *fat cat*

1.   bitter baking staple   _____

2.   10¢ minute   _____

3.   unfalse hint   _____

4.   golf peg charge   _____

5.   messy duplicate   _____

6.   serene tropical tree   _____

7.   unwealthy entryway   _____

8.   frightening small fruit   _____

9.   chilly slobber   _____

10. navy-colored adhesive   _____

11. frozen rain road   _____

12. stressed chain-link   _____

Rhyming Definitions

The answers will be two rhyming words.

Ex.   overweight feline   *fat cat*

1.   shiny evening   _____

2.   inexpensive ewes   _____

3.   conceited locomotive   _____

4.   overly warm small bed   _____

5.   stinky abdomen   _____

6.   tidy chair   _____

7.   sick charcoal cooker   _____

8.   fantasy crew   _____

9.   non-wet pastry   _____

10. sugary 12-inch units   _____

11. artificial serpent   _____

12. crabby kerchief   _____

Rhyming Definitions

The answers will be two rhyming words.

Ex. overweight feline   *fat cat*

1. curly turkey sauce   _____

2. humorous currency   _____

3. greasy lace napkin   _____

4. yearly guidebook   _____

5. superior type of cheese   _____

6. gorilla cloak   _____

7. insect floor mat   _____

8. aching wild pig   _____

9. male sun glow   _____

10. crooked camping shelter   _____

11. uncooked wood-cutting tool   _____

12. candle dripping surcharge   _____

Rhyming Definitions

The answers will be two rhyming words.

Ex.   overweight feline   _____fat cat_____

1.   unintelligent chewing piece   _____

2.   watercraft outerwear   _____

3.   wimpy bird bill   _____

4.   timid winged insect   _____

5.   doe equipment   _____

6.   faithful potting dirt   _____

7.   blaze purchaser   _____

8.   hushed food restriction   _____

9.   courageous whitecap   _____

10. flaking overhead wall   _____

11. strange white fish   _____

12. considerate watermelon peel   _____

Rhyming Definitions

The answers will be two rhyming words.

Ex. overweight feline   *fat cat* _____

1. rodent residence _____

2. heisted intestine _____

3. fractured souvenir _____

4. tiresome linoleum _____

5. envious garden structure _____

6. tanned cowhide, climate _____

7. growing season, bee bite _____

8. margarine, hoarded items _____

9. 8-legged bug, fermented juice _____

10. milking animal, promise _____

11. precipitation, walking stick _____

12. chopped lettuce, sad song _____

Brand Names

Write a specific brand name for each product.

1. soda   _____

2. potato chips   _____

3. candy bar   _____

4. soup   _____

5. snack crackers   _____

6. TV dinner   _____

7. rice   _____

8. bread   _____

9. peanut butter   _____

10. salad dressing   _____

11. ice cream   _____

12. coffee   _____

Brand Names

Write a specific brand name for each product.

1. gum _____

2. cookies _____

3. cereal _____

4. bacon _____

5. frozen pizza _____

6. tea _____

7. pasta sauce _____

8. cheese _____

9. cake mix _____

10. catsup _____

11. jelly _____

12. beer _____

Brand Names

Write a specific brand name for each product.

1. shampoo _____

2. mouthwash _____

3. soap _____

4. razor _____

5. tissues _____

6. toilet paper _____

7. paper towels _____

8. dish soap _____

9. detergent _____

10. diapers _____

11. pain reliever _____

12. cough drops _____

Brand Names

Write a specific brand name for each product.

1. shoes   _____

2. jeans   _____

3. bicycle   _____

4. major appliance   _____

5. automobile   _____

6. airline   _____

7. hotel   _____

8. magazine   _____

9. record label   _____

10. movie studio   _____

11. department store   _____

12. discount store   _____

Famous Names

Write a specific name for each item.

1. actor _____

2. band _____

3. singer _____

4. comedian _____

5. talk show host _____

6. game show host _____

7. TV judge _____

8. reality star _____

9. supermodel _____

10. fashion designer _____

11. chef _____

12. magician _____

Famous Names

Write a specific name for each item.

1. newscaster   _____

2. politician   _____

3. foreign leader   _____

4. business leader   _____

5. fitness guru   _____

6. baseball player   _____

7. basketball player   _____

8. football player   _____

9. tennis player   _____

10. golfer   _____

11. boxer   _____

12. race car driver   _____

Famous Names

Write a specific name for each item.

1. notorious criminal _____

2. Wild West figure _____

3. general _____

4. Native American _____

5. inventor _____

6. composer _____

7. artist _____

8. author _____

9. princess _____

10. king _____

11. Greek god _____

12. fictional monster _____

Famous Names

Write a specific name for each item.

1. fast food mascot   _____

2. nursery rhyme character   _____

3. cartoon character   _____

4. comic strip character   _____

5. dog on film   _____

6. famous cat   _____

7. mountain/range   _____

8. desert   _____

9. forest   _____

10. river   _____

11. ocean   _____

12. beach   _____

Trivia

1. Whose wooden nose grows when he tells a lie?

2. What ship carried the first US settlers?

3. What rag doll has red yarn hair and a triangle nose?

4. What Harlem basketball team traveled the world?

5. What female pilot went missing over the Pacific Ocean?

6. Which fictional detective has a sidekick named Watson?

7. Where does the Pope live?

8. Who is Olive Oyl's sailor boyfriend?

9. What store hosts New York's annual Thanksgiving parade?

10. Who is Batman's sidekick?

11. What tennis tournament is held each July in London?

12. What cartoon character is called "the friendly ghost?"

13. Who is credited with sewing the first American flag?

14. What is the name of Fred Flintstone's wife?

Trivia

1. Who was Fred Astaire's dance partner?

2. Who is credited as the first astronaut to walk on the moon?

3. What is the name of Dorothy's dog in the Wizard of Oz?

4. Who hosted a children's TV show in his "neighborhood?"

5. Which *Happy Days* character wears a leather jacket?

6. What is the name of Elvis Presley's Tennessee mansion?

7. What boxing character was played by Sylvester Stallone?

8. Who developed the theory of relativity and $e=mc^2$?

9. What horse race is held each May at Churchill Downs?

10. What metal toy walks down stairs?

11. Which Jewish girl kept a diary of her life in Nazi Germany?

12. Who "stuck a feather in his cap and called it macaroni"?

13. What 1970's political scandal involved President Nixon?

14. What movie franchise is famous for the phrase, "May the force be with you"?

Trivia

1. Who was raised by apes and married Jane?

2. What famous ship sank in 1912 after hitting an iceberg?

3. Which waterfalls span the US and Canadian border?

4. In movies, what British Secret Service agent goes by 007?

5. What giant lumberjack has a blue ox named Babe?

6. Which civil rights leader refused to give up her bus seat?

7. On what island does the Statue of Liberty stand?

8. Who stole from the rich and gave to the poor?

9. What Parkers Brothers board game features Reading Railroad?

10. What TV family includes Morticia and Uncle Fester?

11. What famous whale bit off Captain Ahab's leg?

12. What company produces popular foam dart guns?

13. Who is Snoopy's bird friend?

14. Who warned, "The British are coming" during his midnight ride?

1. Who broke into the home of the Three Bears?

2. Who invented the telephone?

3. What famous clown had his own TV show?

4. Who wrote "Green Eggs and Ham?"

5. In the fairy tale, who is Hansel's sister?

6. What US harbor was bombed by Japan in 1941?

7. What Muppet frog was the boyfriend of Miss Piggy?

8. In what palace does the Queen of England live?

9. What movie alien wanted to "phone home"?

10. What Scottish body of water is home to Nessie, a sea monster?

11. Where is the New Year's Eve ball dropped in New York City?

12. What Frosted Flakes mascot says, "they're grrrreat?"

13. What region of the Atlantic is known for mysterious disappearances?

14. What McDonald's sandwich has two all-beef patties, special sauce, lettuce, and cheese all on a sesame seed bun?

Rearranging Syllables

Put the syllables in order to form a word.

The first syllable has been underlined.

Ex.: er <u>min</u> al _____mineral_____

1. dant <u>a</u> bun _____

2. pu ter <u>com</u> _____

3. der <u>re</u> main _____

4. bet <u>al</u> pha _____

5. <u>dis</u> sion cus _____

6. mas ja <u>pa</u> _____

7. ty al <u>loy</u> _____

8. liv <u>de</u> er _____

9. ture na <u>sig</u> _____

10. ous er <u>gen</u> _____

11. fact <u>ar</u> ti _____

12. ti <u>spa</u> ghet _____

13. di <u>au</u> ence _____

14. <u>am</u> lance bu _____

Rearranging Syllables

Put the syllables in order to form a word.

The first syllable has been underlined.

Ex.: er <u>min</u> al   <u>   *mineral*   </u>

1.   ee <u>em</u> ploy   _____

2.   na <u>cin</u> mon   _____

3.   <u>re</u> tion flec   _____

4.   late <u>choc</u> o   _____

5.   stru <u>in</u> ment   _____

6.   on ade <u>lem</u>   _____

7.   pin <u>o</u> ion   _____

8.   pi ness <u>hap</u>   _____

9.   tion <u>so</u> lu   _____

10. <u>prin</u> pal ci   _____

11. nym <u>syn</u> o   _____

12. er <u>pro</u> pell   _____

13. u lus <u>stim</u>   _____

14. gna lo <u>bo</u>   _____

Rearranging Syllables	

Put the syllables in order to form a word.

The first syllable has been underlined.

Ex.: er <u>min</u> al   *mineral* _____

1. cue <u>bar</u> be   _____

2. cle <u>re</u> cy   _____

3. <u>pos</u> ble si   _____

4. cro <u>mi</u> wave   _____

5. no <u>dom</u> i   _____

6. er one <u>chap</u>   _____

7. ta to <u>po</u>   _____

8. <u>vic</u> ry to   _____

9. er tom <u>cus</u>   _____

10. <u>lib</u> ty er   _____

11. lope ve <u>en</u>   _____

12. net <u>cab</u> i   _____

13. cate i <u>del</u>   _____

14. <u>cen</u> ry tu   _____

Rearranging Syllables

Put the syllables in order to form a word.

The first syllable has been underlined.

Ex.: er <u>min</u> al   _____mineral_____

1. ni a <u>mac</u> ro   _____

2. de <u>dan</u> on li   _____

3. nol gy o <u>tech</u>   _____

4. ter li cop <u>he</u>   _____

5. sa ver <u>con</u> tion   _____

6. ry go <u>cat</u> e   _____

7. ble vis i <u>in</u>   _____

8. om try e <u>ge</u>   _____

9. le na <u>bal</u> ri   _____

10. do ca <u>a</u> va   _____

11. <u>al</u> na tive ter   _____

12. <u>re</u> ate er frig   _____

13. o dor <u>de</u> ant   _____

14. flow li <u>cau</u> er   _____

Rearranging Syllables

Put the syllables in order to form a word.

The first syllable has been underlined.

Ex.: er <u>min</u> al   *mineral*

1. phy og <u>bi</u> ra   _____

2. <u>dec</u> tion ra o   _____

3. rate <u>e</u> o vap   _____

4. <u>cho</u> ter les ol   _____

5. i tor cal <u>his</u>   _____

6. dil ma lo <u>ar</u>   _____

7. si <u>gym</u> um na   _____

8. <u>ap</u> ate ci pre   _____

9. broi der y <u>em</u>   _____

10. <u>ac</u> di cor on   _____

11. u vid di <u>in</u> al   _____

12. men <u>el</u> e ta ry   _____

13. vi <u>en</u> ment ron al   _____

14. u tions grat la <u>con</u>   _____

Adding Letters

Fill in the missing letters to form words. Answers may vary.

1. b a n d a _ _

2. d e m o l i _ _

3. c l o u _ _

4. h y d r a _ _

5. b o n n _ _

6. r e f l _ _

7. p r o m i _ _

8. s i g _ _

9. g r a v i _ _

10. c i n e _ _

11. c a r o u s _ _

12. i n d _ _

13. k e t t _ _

14. a d m i _ _

15. b r o n _ _

16. h u m b _ _

17. m a g e n _ _

18. c a n v _ _

19. b r o c c o _ _

20. f o s s _ _

21. e m b l _ _

22. c e m e _ _

23. f i b _ _

24. b a s k _ _

25. l u m b _ _

26. c o u p _ _

27. m i l d _ _

28. b r i g _ _

Adding Letters

Fill in the missing letters to form words. Answers may vary.

1. c a b __ __   15. g l o __ __

2. s h r i __ __   16. p l a __ __

3. m a r __ __   17. t r a __ __

4. c l a __ __   18. f l i __ __

5. s c o __ __   19. t h e __ __

6. h u m __ __   20. c a t __ __

7. m u s __ __   21. s t e __ __

8. c r e __ __   22. w o r __ __

9. p l u __ __   23. l a s __ __

10. e x a __ __   24. b l o __ __

11. m o n __ __   25. d r e __ __

12. s p a __ __   26. p h o __ __

13. c o u __ __   27. s w o __ __

14. l e g __ __   28. h o u __ __

Fill in the missing letters to find words. Answers may vary.

1. m o __ __	15. g o __ __
2. c l __ __	16. k n __ __
3. h a __ __	17. s t __ __
4. l o __ __	18. h e __ __
5. s h __ __	19. g l __ __
6. b a __ __	20. p e __ __
7. w h __ __	21. r o __ __
8. p l __ __	22. s p __ __
9. m e __ __	23. f l __ __
10. d u __ __	24. t r __ __
11. o n __ __	25. e d __ __
12. j u __ __	26. w o __ __
13. p a __ __	27. b e __ __
14. d r __ __	28. i n __ __

Adding Letters

Fill in the missing letters to find words. Answers may vary.

1. p i __ __ o w

2. c h __ __ p

3. a u __ __ o r

4. j __ __ g l e

5. q u __ __ t

6. w __ __ d i n g

7. f r __ __ d

8. s p __ __ n

9. f r __ __ h

10. t __ __ t h

11. b l __ __ c h

12. y __ __ l o w

13. h __ __ h

14. b r __ __ d

15. g r __ __ n

16. m __ __ h

17. g __ __ s e

18. s u __ __ e r

19. c r __ __ p

20. p __ __ t y

21. s h __ __ e

22. b __ __ g e

23. p l __ __ e

24. s t __ __ m

25. s h __ __ t

26. b r __ __ e

27. p r __ __ e

28. s p __ __ d

Adding Letters

Fill in the missing letters to find words. Answers may vary.

1. p __ __ c h

2. a l __ __ e

3. c h __ __ e

4. r __ __ c h

5. s m __ __ e

6. t h __ __ e

7. t r __ __ k

8. v i __ __ t

9. s t __ __ e

10. s u __ __ r

11. g u __ __ t

12. l __ __ c h

13. b r __ __ e

14. d r __ __ k

15. s __ __ r

16. m __ __ n

17. c __ __ e

18. b __ __ t

19. w __ __ d

20. r __ __ l

21. d __ __ p

22. f __ __ t

23. g __ __ e

24. l __ __ k

25. t __ __ n

26. p __ __ t

27. d __ __ t

28. s __ __ g

Adding Letters

Fill in the missing letters to find words. Answers may vary.

1. __ __ n s u m e r

2. __ __ z a r d

3. __ __ r t i l l a

4. __ __ o e l a c e

5. __ __ n k r u p t

6. __ __ o r p i o n

7. __ __ a m e t e r

8. __ __ t r i c h

9. __ __ r n a d o

10. __ __ g e l

11. __ __ f f a l o

12. __ __ i m b

13. __ __ a r k

14. __ __ n g r y

15. __ __ t t o o

16. __ __ r a f f e

17. __ __ t t u c e

18. __ __ n o p y

19. __ __ t t r e s s

20. __ __ q u o r

21. __ __ e c k e r s

22. __ __ g i n

23. __ __ f o r d

24. __ __ r r o r

25. __ __ e l t e r

26. __ __ p i r e

27. __ __ b r a r y

28. __ __ r t a i n

Adding Letters

Fill in the missing letters to find words. Answers may vary.

1. _ _ c k e t

2. _ _ l i e f

3. _ _ m m a

4. _ _ n g l e

5. _ _ o w e r

6. _ _ u n k y

7. _ _ i n g

8. _ _ n i s t e r

9. _ _ t i o n

10. _ _ v e r

11. _ _ b b l e

12. _ _ a r e

13. _ _ n d l e

14. _ _ a m e

15. _ _ m e d y

16. _ _ a n t

17. _ _ i c k

18. _ _ a r m

19. _ _ i n k

20. _ _ o v e

21. _ _ i g h t

22. _ _ m b l e

23. _ _ a k e

24. _ _ n n e r

25. _ _ a c k

26. _ _ n g e r

27. _ _ a n k

28. _ _ w n

Fill in the missing letters to find words. Answers may vary.

1. __ __ n d

2. __ __ a w

3. __ __ b e

4. __ __ o k

5. __ __ r n

6. __ __ n e

7. __ __ r e

8. __ __ s t

9. __ __ c e

10. __ __ d e

11. __ __ r d

12. __ __ n g

13. __ __ e d

14. __ __ k e

15. __ __ s e

16. __ __ c h

17. __ __ e e

18. __ __ m e

19. __ __ g e

20. __ __ l l

21. __ __ t h

22. __ __ m p

23. __ __ s s

24. __ __ v e

25. __ __ s h

26. __ __ g s

27. __ __ s p

28. __ __ l p

Completing Roots

Add letters to form words. Answers will vary.

1. be_____

2. be_____

3. be_____

4. be_____

5. be_____

6. be_____

7. be_____

8. be_____

9. be_____

10. be_____

11. so_____

12. so_____

13. so_____

14. so_____

15. so_____

16. so_____

17. so_____

18. so_____

19. so_____

20. so_____

Completing Roots

Add letters to form words. Answers will vary.

1. fr_____

2. fr_____

3. fr_____

4. fr_____

5. fr_____

6. fr_____

7. fr_____

8. fr_____

9. fr_____

10. fr_____

11. di_____

12. di_____

13. di_____

14. di_____

15. di_____

16. di_____

17. di_____

18. di_____

19. di_____

20. di_____

Completing Roots

Add letters to form words. Answers will vary.

1. cr_____

2. cr_____

3. cr_____

4. cr_____

5. cr_____

6. cr_____

7. cr_____

8. cr_____

9. cr_____

10. cr_____

11. th_____

12. th_____

13. th_____

14. th_____

15. th_____

16. th_____

17. th_____

18. th_____

19. th_____

20. th_____

Completing Roots

Add letters to form words. Answers will vary.

1. ma_____

2. ma_____

3. ma_____

4. ma_____

5. ma_____

6. ma_____

7. ma_____

8. ma_____

9. ma_____

10. ma_____

11. wi_____

12. wi_____

13. wi_____

14. wi_____

15. wi_____

16. wi_____

17. wi_____

18. wi_____

19. wi_____

20. wi_____

Completing Roots

Add letters to form words. Answers will vary.

1. pr _____

2. pr _____

3. pr _____

4. pr _____

5. pr _____

6. pr _____

7. pr _____

8. pr _____

9. pr _____

10. pr _____

11. ch_____

12. ch_____

13. ch_____

14. ch_____

15. ch_____

16. ch_____

17. ch_____

18. ch_____

19. ch_____

20. ch _____

Completing Roots

Add letters to form words. Answers will vary.

1. qu _____

2. qu _____

3. qu _____

4. qu _____

5. qu _____

6. qu _____

7. qu _____

8. qu _____

9. qu _____

10. qu _____

11. re_____

12. re_____

13. re _____

14. re_____

15. re_____

16. re_____

17. re_____

18. re_____

19. re_____

20. re_____

Make words of three or more letters from the given word.

W A T E R S L I D E

_____   _____

_____   _____

_____   _____

_____   _____

_____   _____

_____   _____

_____   _____

_____   _____

Reorganizing Words

Make words of three or more letters from the given word.

M A N U S C R I P T

_____   _____

_____   _____

_____   _____

_____   _____

_____   _____

_____   _____

_____   _____

_____   _____

Make words of three or more letters from the given word.

FEATHERBED

_____   _____

_____   _____

_____   _____

_____   _____

_____   _____

_____   _____

_____   _____

_____   _____

Reorganizing Words

Make words of three or more letters from the given word.

QUESTIONABLE

_____   _____

_____   _____

_____   _____

_____   _____

_____   _____

_____   _____

_____   _____

_____   _____

Make words of three or more letters from the given word.

L U M B E R J A C K

_____   _____

_____   _____

_____   _____

_____   _____

_____   _____

_____   _____

_____   _____

_____   _____

Personalized Pages

Think of a hobby that interests you and write it below.	Think of your favorite holiday and write it below.
_____	_____
List words associated with that hobby.	List words associated with that holiday.
_____	_____
_____	_____
_____	_____
_____	_____
_____	_____
_____	_____
_____	_____

Personalized Pages

Think of a travel destination and write it below.

_____

List words associated with that location.

_____

_____

_____

_____

_____

_____

_____

Think of a person in your life and write is or her name below.

_____

List words to describe that person.

_____

_____

_____

_____

_____

_____

_____

Personalized Pages

Write the name of the city where you live.	
Using the city above, list cities nearby.	Using the city above, list area attractions.

Personalized Pages

Write the name of your favorite restaurant	
Using the restaurant above, list items on the menu.	Using the restaurant above, list places nearby.

Personalized Pages

Think of your favorite month and write it below.

[   ]

Using the word in the box, think of a word in each category that starts with the same (**first letter.**)

person   _____

place   _____

thing   _____

action   _____

description   _____

Using the word in the box, think of a word in each category that starts with the same (**last letter.**)

person   _____

place   _____

thing   _____

action   _____

description   _____

Personalized Pages

Think of your favorite season and write it below.

[   ]

Using the word in the box, think of a word in each category that starts with the same (**first letter.**)

person   _____

place   _____

thing   _____

action   _____

description   _____

Using the word in the box, think of a word in each category that starts with the same (**last letter.**)

person   _____

place   _____

thing   _____

action   _____

description   _____

Personalized Pages

Think of your favorite type of weather and write it below.

Using the word in the box, think of a word in each category that starts with the same (**first letter.**)

person   _____

place   _____

thing   _____

action   _____

description   _____

Using the word in the box, think of a word in each category that starts with the same (**last letter.**)

person   _____

place   _____

thing   _____

action   _____

description   _____

Personalized Pages

Think of a color you like and write it below.

Think of words that start with the same (first letter.)

_____   _____

_____   _____

_____   _____

_____   _____

_____   _____

_____   _____

_____   _____

Personalized Pages

Think of a sound you like and write it below.

Think of words that start with the same (first letter.)

_____   _____

_____   _____

_____   _____

_____   _____

_____   _____

_____   _____

_____   _____

Personalized Pages

Think of a scent you like and write it below.

Think of words that start with the same (first letter.)

_____   _____

_____   _____

_____   _____

_____   _____

_____   _____

_____   _____

_____   _____

_____   _____

Print your full name below.

_____

Using the letters above, make words of 3 or more letters.

_____

_____

_____

_____

_____

_____

_____

_____

Print your birth city and state below.

_____

Using the letters above, make words of 3 or more letters.

_____

_____

_____

_____

_____

_____

_____

_____

KEY

This key includes examples of correct answers.
You may come up with other appropriate responses.

ASSOCIATED FILL-INS

Page 7 CAMPING: backpack, tent, stars, firewood, ranger, campsite, lantern, compass, sleeping bag, s'mores, binoculars, cabin, hammock, bonfire

Page 8 FISHING: pole, bait/boat, bobber, hook, sinker, net, tackle box, lure, reel, waders, cast, river, deep-sea, rod

Page 9 BOOKS: title, hardcover, chapter, pages, biography, bookmark, cover, illustrator, publisher, fiction, bookworm, paperback, library, author

Page 10 TRAVEL: luggage, vacation, road trip, reservation, travel agent, sightseeing, passport, rest stop, hotel, destination, resort, airplane, cruise ship, tourist

Page 11 MONEY: dollar, deposit, change jar, bonds, interest, stockbroker, money order, debit card, transfer, checking account, withdrawal, budget, savings, wealthy

Page 12 WEATHER: sunny, thunderstorm, warm breeze, forecast, humidity, drizzle, temperature, tornado, climate change, snow flurries, jet stream, blizzard, precipitation, meteorologist

WORD DEDUCTION

Page 13 giraffe, shovel, spoon, dice, salad, web, yolk, razor, tricycle, curtain, axe, banana, penguin, purr, picnic

Page 14 syrup, wings, whistle, octopus, floss, cane, vacuum, crust, dozen, attic, skunk, leash, grill, piano, hose

Page 15 eraser, cactus, shell, paint, crown, tattoo, porcupine, diamond, pouch, cashier, statue, camel, dugout, magnet, vitamin

Page 16 pillow, bubble, plow, chimney, allowance, collar, armor, arch, bleach, cart, snore, balloon, pilot, dictionary, anniversary

Page 17 taxi, flag, aisle, throne, lava, scholarship, yoga, litter, aluminum, caffeine, dentures, venom, hurricane, blade, dribble

WORDS THAT FOLLOW (answers may vary)

Page 18 hot cocoa/hot dog, shopping bag/shopping cart, sweet tooth/sweetheart, bookmark/book bag, dishrag/dish soap, goodbye/good luck, tea bag/teacup, chicken soup/chicken breast, seashell/seaweed, mailbox/mail carrier, toothache/tooth fairy, raincoat/rainbow, vanilla ice cream/vanilla pudding, beach ball/beach umbrella

Page 19 ice cream/ice cube, fried chicken/fried rice, lucky charm/lucky duck, weatherproof/weathervane, eyeball/eyelash, water fountain/waterfall, car keys/car wash, tomato sauce/tomato paste, bathrobe/bathmat, coffeepot/coffee cup, silver lining/silver dollar, heartbeat/heartache, fortune teller/fortune cookie, apple pie/apple cider

Page 20 best man/best friend, tree trunk/tree house, pork loin/pork chop, sandbox/sandcastle, snowball/snowman, shredded cheese/shredded wheat, window washer/window seat, night light/nightfall, potato chip/potato salad, salad dressing/salad bar, haircut/hairbrush, pillowcase/pillow fight, gold ring/gold rush, hula hoop/hula dancer

Page 21 birdhouse/birdbath, honeybee/honeycomb, cotton candy/cotton ball, life jacket/lifestyle, lunch hour/lunchbox, gift card/gift bag, windmill/windchime, houseboat/house guest, earwax/earmuffs, dirty dishes/dirty laundry, middleman/middle class, rocking chair/rocking horse, sunshine/sunglasses, belly button/bellyache

LISTING ASSOCIATED WORDS (answers may vary)

Page 22 THE FOREST: trails, trees, leaves, mushrooms, moss, birds, fox, deer, bugs **A FARM:** farmer, tractor, barn, silo, crops, chickens, pigs, cows, horses **THE BEACH:** sand, ocean, waves, seagulls, seashells, sandcastles, beach umbrellas, sunbathers, lifeguard
Page 23 A BASEBALL GAME: pitcher, catcher, umpire, baseball, bat, bases, uniforms, hot dogs, peanuts **A WEDDING:** bride, groom, minister, flower girl, ring bearer, photographer, dresses, rings, bouquet
A CIRCUS: big-top, ringmaster, clowns, kids, tightrope, trapeze, lions, tigers, bears

Key

Page 24 A SCHOOL: principal, teachers, students, chalkboard, globe, desks, lockers, book bags, pencils **AN AIRPORT:** security, boarding pass, pilot, flight attendant, travelers, luggage, passport, runway, plane
A NURSERY: crib, mobile, blanket, stuffed animals, changing table, diaper pail, diapers, rocking chair, board books

SCRAMBLED CATEGORIES

Page 25 TYPES OF BREAD: rye, whole wheat, pita, corn, pumpernickel, banana, sourdough **TYPES OF CAKE:** fruitcake, red velvet, angel food, chocolate, cheesecake, carrot, lemon

Page 26 TYPES OF MUSIC: jazz, disco, rock and roll, folk, country, hip hop, classical **TYPES OF DANCE:** tap, ballroom, ballet, polka, can-can, tango, Hokey Pokey

Page 27 TYPES OF SHOES: penny loafer, clog, sandal, sneaker, flip-flop, high heel, cowboy boot **TYPES OF FABRIC:** silk, wool, canvas, burlap, nylon, cotton, polyester

Page 28 TYPES OF TRUCKS: semi, dump, tow, cement, garbage, pickup, delivery **TYPES OF BOATS:** tugboat, canoe, yacht, sailboat, ferry, speedboat, barge

Page 29 COUNTRIES: Ireland, Brazil, Morocco, Norway, Poland, Switzerland, Egypt **LANGUAGES:** Italian, French, English, Portuguese, Greek, Chinese, Sign Language

Page 30 PLANETS: Mercury, Venus, Earth, Jupiter, Neptune, Saturn, Mars **TABLE OF ELEMENTS:** copper, carbon, nitrogen, sodium, oxygen, iron, hydrogen

Key

CATEGORIES A-Z (answers may vary)

Page 31 ANIMALS: antelope, bear, cat, dog, elephant, fish, gorilla, hyena, iguana, jaguar, kangaroo, lion, monkey, newt, octopus, pig, quail, rabbit, snake, turtle, vulture, whale, yak, zebra

Page 32 FOODS: apple, biscuit, carrot, doughnut, egg, fish, grilled cheese, hamburger, ice cream, jelly, kale, lasagna, macaroni, noodles, oatmeal, pancake, quesadilla, rice, soup, taco, veal, waffle, yogurt

Page 33 WOMEN'S NAMES: Ann, Becky, Carrie, Diane, Ellen, Frances, Ginger, Helen, Isabelle, Jill, Kim, Lilly, Monica, Nicole, Olive, Patty, Rose, Stacy, Tonya, Violet, Wanda, Yolanda

Page 34 MEN'S NAMES: Adam, Bob, Charlie, David, Ed, Frank, Gary, Hank, Isaac, Jack, Ken, Luke, Matt, Neil, Oscar, Paul, Quinton, Randy, Sam, Tom, Victor, Walter, Zach

CATEGORIES BY LETTER (answers may vary)

Page 35 A: Austin (TX), Alabama, Argentina, art, accountant, ankle, aspen, asparagus, almond, apple **B:** Boston (MA), biology, brakes, beagle, bass, bridge, basketball, broccoli, bagel, blueberry

Page 36 C: Chicago (IL), collie, canary, catfish, carnation, coffee, cashew, cumin, cherry, chocolate **D:** Detroit (MI), Delaware, Denmark, dentist, dalmatian, dogwood, daisy, diamond, doughnut, dill

Page 37 E: El Paso (TX), England, electrician, elbow, engine, eagle, eel, elm, emerald, eggplant **F:** Fargo (ND), Florida, Finland, Father's Day, firefighter, finger, fender, flamingo, flounder, football

Key

Page 38 G: Georgia, Greece, geography, gardener, gums, golden retriever, goldfish, golf, grapes, ginger **H:** Honolulu (HI), Hawaii, Holland, history, hairdresser, hood, hummingbird, hockey, harp, hazelnut

Page 39 I: Indianapolis (IN), Iowa, Italy, indigo, inspector, intestine, ignition, iris, iced tea, ice cream **K:** Kalamazoo (MI), Kentucky, Kenya, khaki, knee, karate, kazoo, Kings in the Corner, kiwi, kale

Page 40 L: Las Vegas (NV), Louisiana, Labor Day, lavender, lawyer, Labrador retriever, lilac, lemon, lettuce, lemonade **M:** Mobile (AL), Maine, Mother's Day, maroon, model, minnow, mum, mango, macadamia, mint chocolate chip

Page 41 N: New Orleans (LA), Nebraska, Nepal, New Year's Eve, navy blue, nurse, nose, nectarine, nutmeg, Neapolitan **O:** Omaha (NE), Oklahoma, optometrist, owl, oak, opal, oboe, orange, onion, oatmeal

Page 42 P: poodle, peacock, pine, pearl, piano, poker, pancake, peanut, paprika, pumpkin **R:** Rhode Island, realtor, robin, redwood, rose, ruby, rummy, raspberry, radish, root beer

Page 43 S: South Dakota, science, surgeon, Saint Bernard, sparrow, sunflower, soccer, saxophone, solitaire, strawberry **T:** Toledo (OH), Tennessee, Thanksgiving, tan, teacher, toe, tire, terrier, turkey, turmeric

Page 44 V: Venice (FL), Virginia, Vietnam, Valentine's Day, veterinarian, vulture, violet, volleyball, violin, vanilla **W:** Walla Walla (WA), Wyoming, waiter, wrist, windshield wipers, woodpecker, willow, watermelon, waffle, walnut

LISTING CATEGORY MEMBERS (answers may vary)

Page 45 THINGS THAT ARE GREEN: grass, leaves, hose, alligator, frog, dollar, peas, broccoli **THINGS THAT ARE YELLOW:** sun, yield sign, school bus, daffodil, pencil, mustard, banana, lemon

Page 46 KITCHEN UTENSILS: can opener, measuring cups, knife, whisk, spatula, tongs, grater, peeler **SWEET TREATS:** cookies, brownies, cake, pie, ice cream, pudding, fudge, candy

Page 47 TOOLS: hammer, axe, wrench, screwdriver, pliers, saw, drill, ruler **BUGS:** bee, ladybug, beetle, fly, firefly, ant, mosquito, cockroach

Page 48 SPORTS TEAMS: New York Yankees, Boston Red Sox, St. Louis Cardinals, LA Dodgers, Chicago Bears, New England Patriots, Green Bay Packers, Dallas Cowboys **FAMOUS LANDMARKS:** Statue of Liberty, Empire State Building, Mt. Rushmore, Golden Gate Bridge, Grand Canyon, Eiffel Tower, Taj Mahal, Stonehenge

BEGINS WITH

Page 49 A: anchor, actor, apron, album, acorn, applause, acrobat, ashes, absent, accelerator, agriculture, admire, alarm, aroma

Page 50 B: blink, broom, bracelet, bachelor, bitter, beverage, belch, bilingual, bale, brunette, brew, ballot, boomerang, balance

Page 51 C: comb, crayon, curb, caboose, comedian, cone, catalog, confident, crumb, cancel, commute, cockpit, coupon, cast

Page 52 D: dynamite, disappear, deputy, decade, dam, digest, dungeon, donate, detour, dormitory, deal, diary, dragon, deli

Page 53 E: echo, elope, escalator, enter, eerie, enroll, extinct, edible, eavesdrop, election, exhale, error, escape, entrée

Page 54 F: freckles, fever, flash, favorite, fetch, fracture, faucet, frequent, fumble, familiar, fasten, furnace, fugitive, foul

Page 55 G: gulp, guard, gamble, gallery, gobble, guest, generic, giggle, guarantee, globe, genie, goal, gust, grammar

Page 56 H: hoof, history, hamper, honest, hum, harbor, habit, halo, hive, humble, hibernate, hinge, hut, hurdle

Page 57 I: indigo, illegal, immune, index, inflate, imitate, igloo, ignite, income, innocent, identical, ignore, imposter, ivory

Page 58 J: jacket, juggle, jerky, joke, jet, jeans, jury, jungle, jaguar, jealous, joker, jog, juvenile, jukebox

Page 59 K: kindergarten, karate, kite, kilt, kidneys, koala, kayak, keg, kettle, kennel, kernel, keyboard, kerosene, knuckles

Page 60 L: limousine, licorice, lazy, lyrics, leak, ladle, lobby, lasso, loan, logo, launch, lard, lather, lullaby

Page 61 M: mustache, menu, measure, mitt, marble, mayor, mural, massage, manure, mob, marinate, matinee, mall, mist

Page 62 N: noisy, nachos, neon, net, nanny, narrow, nightmare, nibble, neutral, nugget, noodles, numb, nominate, nectar

Page 63 O: oath, oval, office, odor, obvious, ostrich, ointment, obese, opera, original, orchestra, organs, orchard, optimist

Page 64 P: puddle, palace, prune, pigeon, paddle, perfume, polish, prison, pickle, pollen, pierce, parka, peel, pinch

Page 65 Q: quit, quail, question, quart, quench, queasy, quiz, quarantine, quilt, quiche, quarterly, quake, quote, quaint

Page 66 R: racket, repair, rattle, reptile, rehearse, rotten, rash, rescue, rifle, recipe, reunion, rinse, resume, robe

Page 67 S: schedule, scarf, skillet, silence, safari, swamp, sandpaper, semester, steam, salary, scar, sample, shingles, sling

Page 68 T: tear, tavern, thaw, tattle, talent, tank, tile, toupee, toddler, trophy, traffic, tuxedo, tobacco, testimony

Page 69 U: utensil, umpire, urgent, uniform, understand, usher, universe, ukulele, university, umbrella, utopia, unique, upholster, unanimous

Page 70 V: vision, velvet, village, volume, valedictorian, veil, vain, valet, varnish, vinegar, verdict, vertebrae, vending, veto

Page 71 W: whisper, wardrobe, wand, wrench, waste, warehouse, whisk, wound, waltz, wilt, warrant, wreath, wisdom, wade

Page 72 Y: yam, yeast, yarn, yardstick, yank, yak, yield, Yeti, yearly, yogurt, youth, yearn, yap, yodel

Page 73 Z: zucchini, Zen, zit, zipper, zinc, zinnia, zoology, zipline, zigzag, zone, zodiac, zero, ziplock, zany

WH- DEFINITIONS

Page 74 bib, luau, wick, shin, submarine, suspenders, puppet, pulse, knot, gravel, beak, diploma, avalanche, carton

Page 75 helmet, fountain, vest, batter, petals, logs, auction, antenna, appetite, calculator, thermos, starch, gravity, combination

Page 76 captain, barber, DJ, pharmacist, accountant, chauffeur, principal, tour guide, seamstress/tailor, tutor, jockey, lifeguard, athlete, substitute

Page 77 florist, realtor, janitor, dermatologist, illustrator, architect, conductor, volunteer, exterminator, chiropractor, miner, entrepreneur, choreographer, caterer

Page 78 cafeteria, pantry, shelter, courtroom, laundromat, auditorium, circus, vault, laboratory, casino, stable, theater, aquarium, stadium

Page 79 studio, factory, locker-room, cellar, bakery, greenhouse, groomer, campground, coop, rink, poll, hangar, silo, arcade

DOUBLE DEFINITIONS

Page 80 club, rock, file, bark, trip, date, play, ring, iron, can, row, patient

Page 81 change, stall, remote, right, pound, hide, park, roll, wave, box, bow, pitch

Page 82 palm, mine, tie, brush, light, watch, key, serve, second, tire, branch, degree

Page 83 jam, chip, train, spoke, bear, suit, mint, current, fall, scale, ruler, fan

Page 84 top, fire, bank, sink, board, seal, duck, staff, bore, novel, stalk, mole

COMPOUND DEFINITIONS

Page 85 upbeat, nightgown, gumdrop, eggplant, milkshake, rainbow, honeydew, moonshine

Page 86 wishbone, roughhouse, heartburn, offspring, bigwig, billboard, wintergreen, frostbite

Page 87 flapjack, drawbridge, centerpiece, breakfast, needlepoint, cargo, toadstool, hopscotch

Page 88 popcorn, blueprint, cheapskate, carpool, potpie, hushpuppy, invoice, jigsaw

Page 89 quarterback, bedspread, aftermath, hedgehog, trademark, undercarriage, forecast, landlord

Page 90 candlelight, heirloom, stalemate, potluck, shuffleboard, scarecrow, patchwork, stagecoach

RHYMING DEFINITIONS

Page 91 old mold, blue shoe, free tree, fun nun, slow crow, cold gold, damp lamp, clean queen, dark bark, quick lick, real seal, red bed

Page 92 sour flour, dime time, true clue, tee fee, sloppy copy, calm palm, poor door, scary berry, cool drool, blue glue, sleet street, tense fence

Page 93 bright night, cheap sheep, vain train, hot cot, smelly belly, neat seat, ill grill, dream team, dry pie, sweet feet, fake snake, cranky hankie

Page 94 wavy gravy, funny money, oily doily, annual manual, better cheddar, ape cape, bug rug, sore boar, man tan, bent tent, raw saw, wax tax

Page 95 dumb gum, boat coat, weak beak, shy fly, dear gear, loyal soil, fire buyer, quiet diet, brave wave, peeling ceiling, odd cod, kind rind

Page 96 mouse house, stolen colon, broken token, boring flooring, jealous trellis, leather weather, spring sting, butter clutter, spider cider, cow vow, rain cane, salad ballad

BRAND NAMES (answers may vary)

Page 97 Coca-Cola, Pringles, Hershey, Campbell's, Ritz, Swanson, Rice A Roni, Wonder, Jif, Hidden Valley, Breyers, Folgers

Page 98 Wrigley, Oreo, Kellogg's, Oscar Mayer, Tombstone, Lipton, Prego, Kraft, Betty Crocker, Heinz, Smucker's, Budweiser

Page 99 Head & Shoulders, Listerine, Dove, Bic, Puffs, Charmin, Bounty, Palmolive, Tide, Pampers, Tylenol, Halls

Page 100 Nike, Levi's, Schwinn, Maytag, Chevrolet, United, Hilton, Time, RCA, MGM, Macy's, Dollar Tree

FAMOUS NAMES (answers may vary)

Page 101 Jack Nicholson, The Beatles, Frank Sinatra, Eddie Murphy, Oprah Winfrey, Bob Barker, Judge Judy, Kim Kardashian, Cindy Crawford, Calvin Klein, Julia Child, David Copperfield

Page 102 Barbara Walters, John F. Kennedy, Nelson Mandela, Bill Gates, Richard Simmons, Jackie Robinson, Michael Jordan, Walter Payton, John McEnroe, Tiger Woods, Muhammad Ali, Dale Earnhardt

Page 103 Al Capone, Annie Oakley, Robert E. Lee, Sitting Bull, Thomas Edison, Ludwig van Beethoven, Leonardo Da Vinci, Mark Twain, Princess Diana, King Tut, Zeus, Godzilla

Page 104 Ronald McDonald, Humpty Dumpty, Bugs Bunny, Blondie, Lassie, Garfield, Rocky Mountains, Sahara Desert, Redwood Forest, Mississippi River, Pacific Ocean, Waikiki Beach

TRIVIA

Page 105 Pinocchio, Mayflower, Raggedy Ann, Harlem Globetrotters, Amelia Earhart, Sherlock Holmes, Vatican, Popeye, Macy's, Robin, Wimbledon, Casper, Betsy Ross, Wilma

Page 106 Ginger Rogers, Neil Armstrong, Toto, Mr. Rogers, Fonzie, Graceland, Rocky, Albert Einstein, Kentucky Derby, Slinky, Anne Frank, Yankee Doodle, Watergate, Star Wars

Page 107 Tarzan, Titanic, Niagara Falls, James Bond, Paul Bunyan, Rosa Parks, Ellis Island, Robin Hood, Monopoly, Addams Family, Moby Dick, Nerf, Woodstock, Paul Revere

Page 108 Goldilocks, Alexander Bell, Bozo, Dr. Seuss, Gretel, Pearl Harbor, Kermit, Buckingham Palace, ET, Loch Ness, Times Square, Tony the Tiger, Bermuda Triangle, Big Mac

REARRANGING SYLLABLES

Page 109 abundant, computer, remainder, alphabet, discussion, pajamas, loyalty, deliver, signature, generous, artifact, spaghetti, audience, ambulance

Page 110 employee, cinnamon, reflection, chocolate, instrument, lemonade, opinion, happiness, solution, principal, synonym, propeller, stimulus, bologna

Page 111 barbecue, recycle, possible, microwave, domino, chaperone, potato, victory, customer, liberty, envelope, cabinet, delicate, century

Page 112 macaroni, dandelion, technology, helicopter, conversation, category, invisible, geometry, ballerina, avocado, alternative, refrigerate, deodorant, cauliflower

Page 113 biography, decoration, evaporate, cholesterol, historical, armadillo, gymnasium, appreciate, embroidery, accordion, individual, elementary, environmental, congratulations

ADDING LETTERS (answers may vary)

Page 114 bandana, demolish, cloudy, hydrant, bonnet, reflex, promise, sight, gravity, cinema, carousel, index, kettle, admire **/** bronze, humble, magenta, canvas, broccoli, fossil, emblem, cement, fiber, basket, lumber, couple, mildew, bright

Page 115 cabin, shrimp, march, class, score, humid, music, creak, plump, exact, money, spark, cough, legal / glory, plain, trail, flirt, these, catch, steak, worse, lasso, block, dread, phone, sword, house

Page 116 more, clue, have, lose, show, band, what, play, meal, dust, only, jump, park, drum / gold, knee, star, hear, glue, pest, rope, spin, flow, tree, edge, work, belt, inch

Page 117 pillow, champ, author, jungle, quiet, wedding, fried, spoon, fresh, tooth, bleach, yellow, high, bread / green, moth, goose, summer, creep, party, shine, barge, plane, steam, short, breeze, pride, speed

Page 118 peach, alive, chore, ranch, smoke, three, truck, visit, stove, sugar, guilt, lunch, broke, drink / sour, moon, care, beet, word, roll, deep, foot, give, link, town, plot, dirt, sing

Page 119 consumer, lizard, tortilla, shoelace, bankrupt, scorpion, diameter, ostrich, tornado, angel, buffalo, climb, shark, hungry / tattoo, giraffe, lettuce, canopy, mattress, liquor, checkers, begin, afford, mirror, shelter, empire, library, curtain

Page 120 pocket, belief, comma, single, flower, chunky, thing, canister, lotion, cover, bubble, share, candle, shame / comedy, grant, stick, charm, blink, glove, bright, gamble, brake, winner, crack, danger, thank, gown

Page 121 hand, draw, cube, book, horn, cane, rare, best, dice, hide, card, king, shed, cake / hose, each, free, game, page, pull, with, lump, mess, love, wish, hugs wasp, gulp

COMPLETING ROOTS (answers may vary)

Page 122 bed, bee, beg, bet, beet, bear, bell, best, better, belly **/**son, song, sock, soft, some, sore, soggy, soup, soap, sofa

Page 123 fry, frame, free, fresh, friend, from, frog, freedom, freeze, fruit **/** did, dig, dime, dip, dial, dice, dish, dinner, diamond, dictionary

Page 124 cry, crab, craft, crash, crawl, cream, creek, crow, crown, crust **/** the, them, they, this, thief, throw, thank, thumb, three, thunder

Page 125 mad, man, map, math, maybe, mama, machine, master, magazine, marshmallow **/** wig, win, wink, with, will, willow, wide, wise, wish, window

Page 126 pray, prize, prison, pride, press, pretty, prince, print, prune, president **/** chin, chip, chop, chain, cheek, chair, chest, child, cheese, chill

Page 127 quit, quiet, quite, quart, quick, quiz, queen, question, quilt, quarter**/** red, read, real, reach, rent, rest, relax, recycle, rebate, refrigerator

REARRANGING WORDS (answers may vary)

Page 128 WATERSLIDE: water, slide, war, was, wet, west, ate, eat, tea, raw, saw, sit, see, sew, let, law, lid, slid, dew, draw

Page 129 MANUSCRIPT: man, map, mat, ant, nut, sun, sat, can, cap, cat, cup, ram, run, pan, pin, pat, pit, put, rain, tuna

Page 130 FEATHERBED: feather, bed, feed, feet, bee, the, hat, her, head, rat, raft, red, read, bread, beat, bear, beef, beet, bath, deer

Page 131 QUESTIONABLE: quest, question, able, quit, set, son, sale, tin, ton, tan, tab, tone, stone, table, stable, nest, nail, bat, bet, best

Page 132 LUMBERJACK: lumber, jack, back, rack, luck, buck, lamb, blue, rum, rub, jam, male, car, care, cake, make, bake, rake, lake, leak

www.ingramcontent.com/pod-product-compliance
Lightning Source LLC
Chambersburg PA
CBHW080017280326

41934CB00015B/3377